Improve Your Sex Life
with Exercise

Improve Your Sex Life with Exercise

H.J. Maxwell

To order additional copies of this book, contact:
Xlibris
1-888-795-4274
www.Xlibris.com
Orders@Xlibris.com
791864

Foreword

Throughout history men have struggled with the problem of impotency or a poor erection. Of course the women in their lives are affected likewise. Good nutrition and exercise are important to our overall well being. However, these are not the only factors necessary for most men to have a great sex life. I have designed an exercise program that will exercise the penis as you would any other area of the body. The program also has the added benefit of instilling a sense of self-confidence in our ability to perform well sexually.

Introduction

Muscle increases in size when exercised. The penis is a mass of thin superficial muscles. The following exercises will strengthen and stretch the muscles, and improve circulation. The result can be a greatly improved erection, with some increase in size. A ten minute workout three days a week can have a significant effect on the ability to obtain a good erection. The exercises can be done more often, if the stretching exercises are alternated with the strengthening exercises. As with any exercise program, proper rest is important to allow muscles time to repair and rebuild. Caution should be taken not to injure or bruise the penis. Start out gently and work up to an application of force that feels right for you. Exercising the penis immediately before sexual intercourse has the added benefit of improving your erection at that time. Some of the exercises are primarily stretching exercises, which involves stretching the muscle fiber under the skin. Other exercises are primarily strengthening, and secondarily stretching. The are many variation of the exercises, limited only by your imagination. Concentrate on contracting the area of the penis between one hand and the other hand. In the beginning, when the muscles are weak, the maximum contraction that can be achieved will not be great. This will improve with time.

Nutrition

Proper nutrition is important in achieving and maintaining a healthy sex life. A well balanced diet of protein, carbohydrates, and fats forms the foundation. Maintain three to four servings a day of protein at all times. Cut back on carbohydrates and fats when you are trying to lose body fat. Supplements are good for added nutrition. The mineral zinc has been shown to increase the testosterone level. Drink plenty of water and try to get three to four servings of fruits and vegetables per day. Micro- nutrients from fruits and vegetables are now available in capsule form, Hold alcohol consumption down to a moderate level. Avoid nicotine for your own health and those around you.

Exercise for the body

Proper exercise of the body contributes to your physical, mental, and emotional well- being. Stretching, strength training, and aerobics are all important. I like to do a series of ten second stretches for versatility. With this method I am also able to get in a large variety of exercises in fifteen to twenty minutes. Strength training is a must for good health as we get older. The back must be kept strong and flexible in order to maintain vitality. The back supports the spine, which is an extension of the brain. I prefer dumbbells to start with because they are so versatile. Barbells and machines are a nice addition to your exercise program. Two to three minutes of stretching is a great way to relieve stress at the end of the day, and can add a great deal to your sex life.

Hold the penis with both hands and contract the penis using the weight to enhance the effect of the exercises.

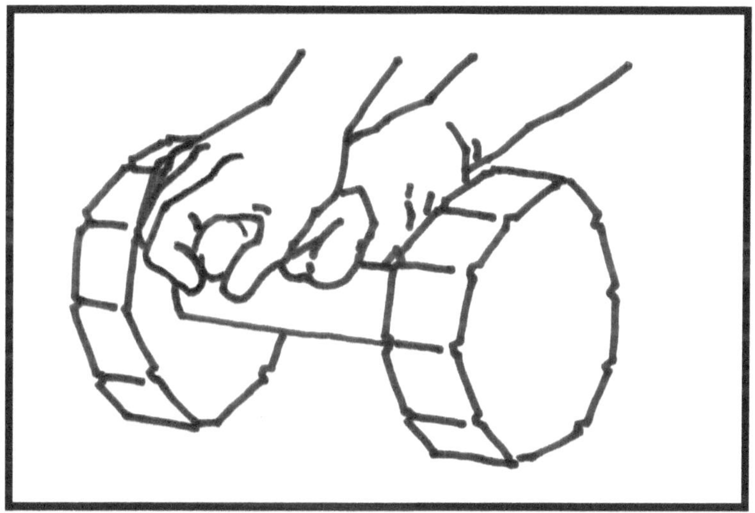

Same procedure, however rotate the penis upside down.

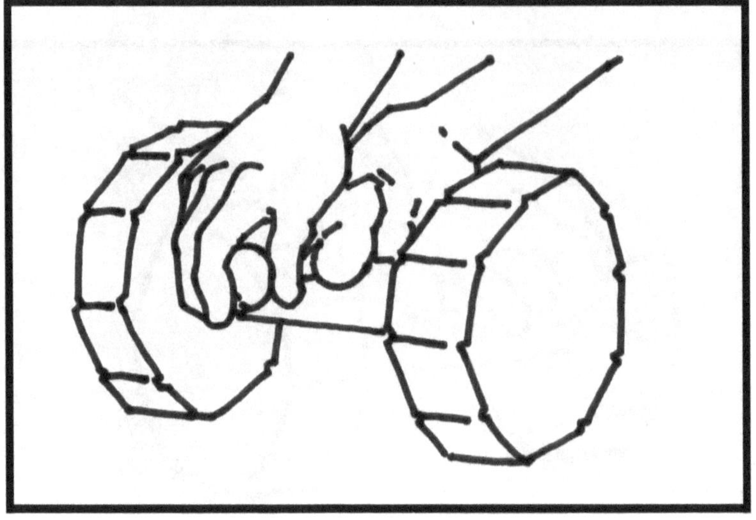

Same procedure, however rotate the penis to the side.

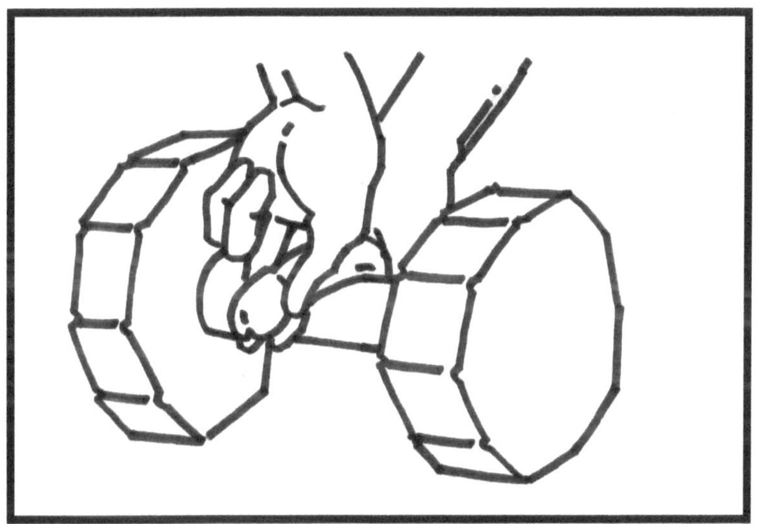

Same procedure, however rotate the penis to the other side.

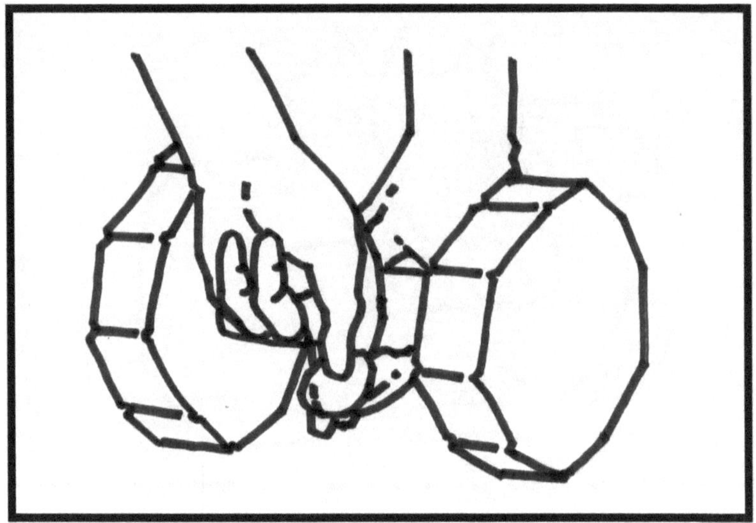

Same procedure, however rotate the penis to the other side.

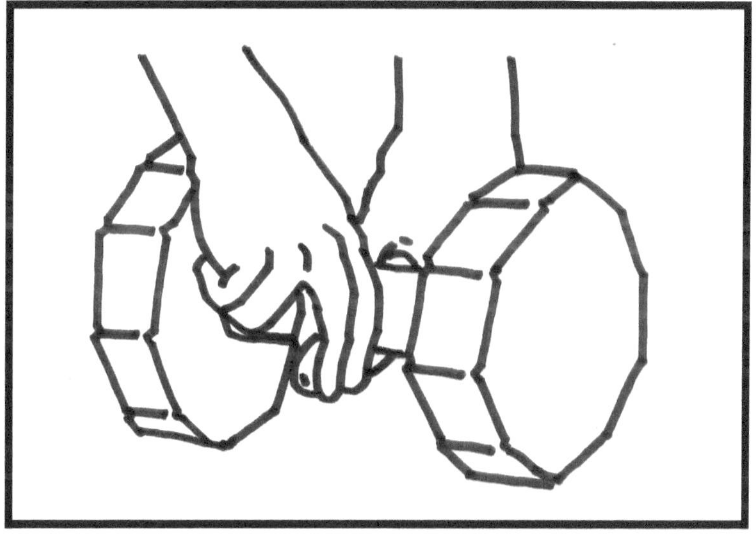

Same procedure, however rotate the penis upside down.

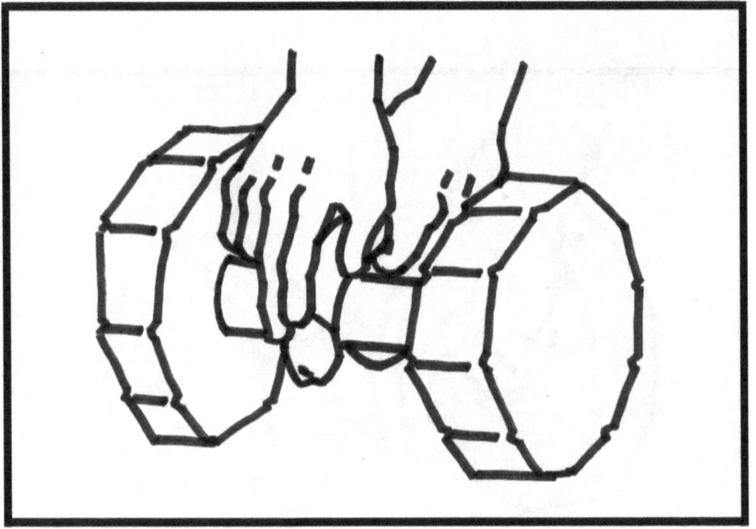

Same procedure, however rotate the penis to the side.

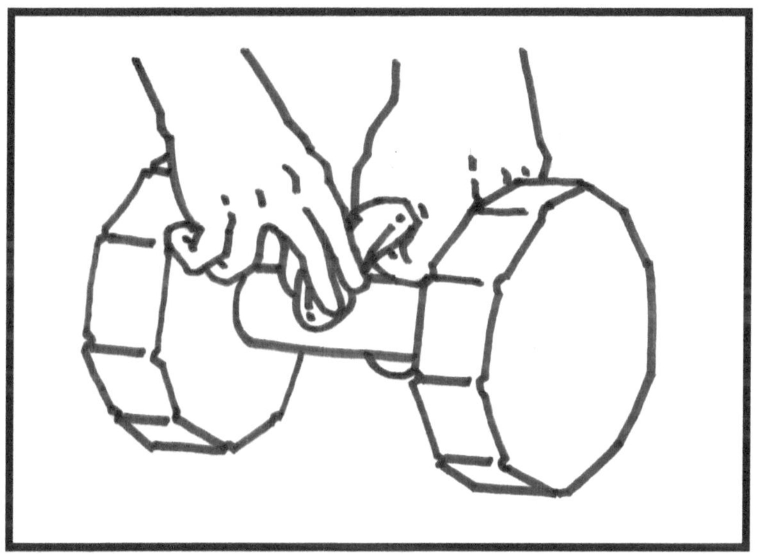

Same procedure, however rotate the penis to the other side.

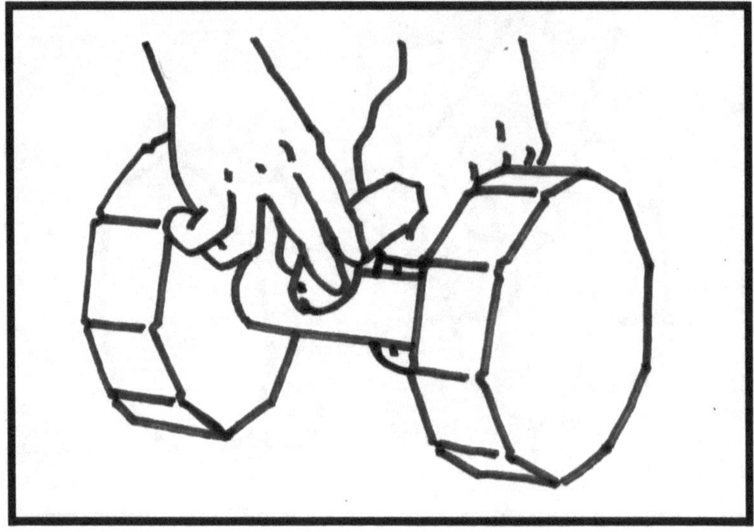

Same procedure, however rotate the penis to the other side.

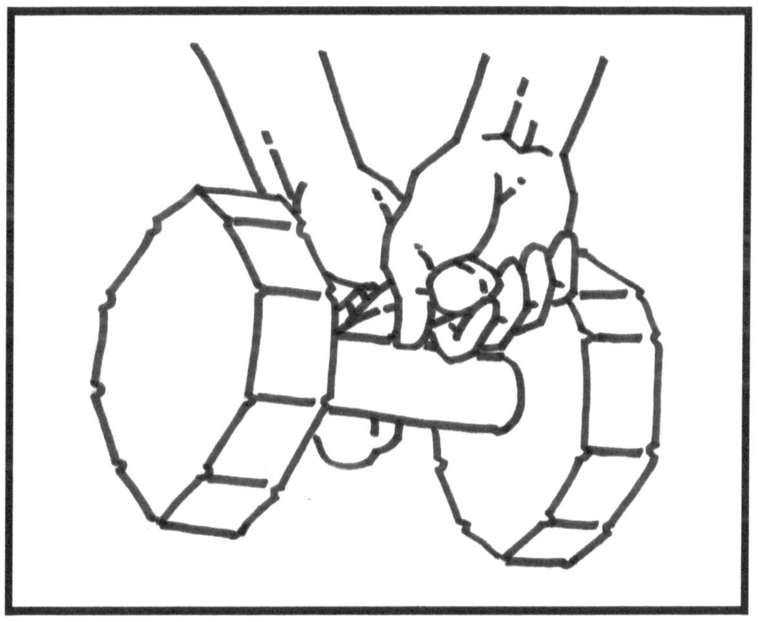

Same procedure, however rotate the penis upside down.

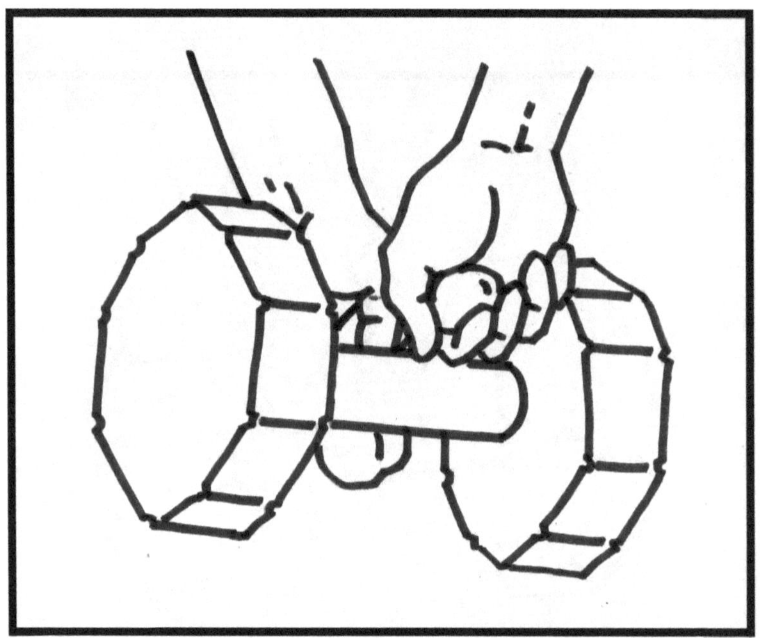

Same procedure, however rotate the penis to the side.

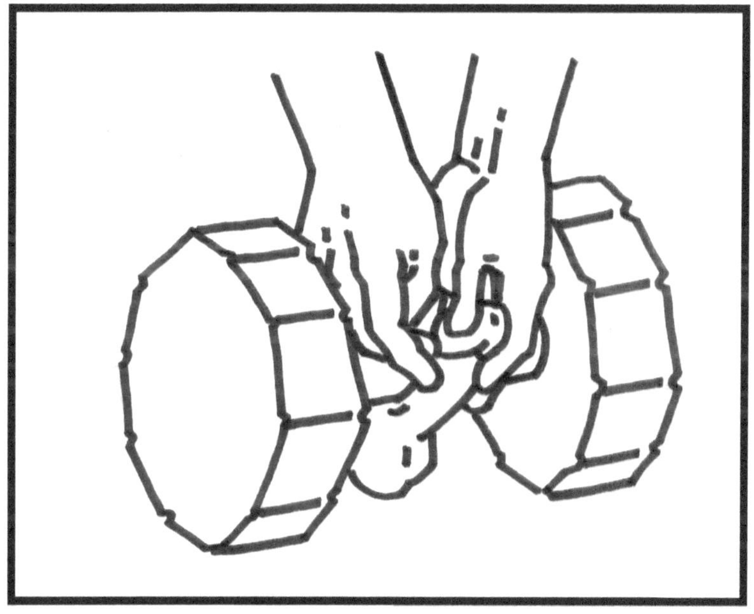

Same procedure, however rotate the penis to the other side.

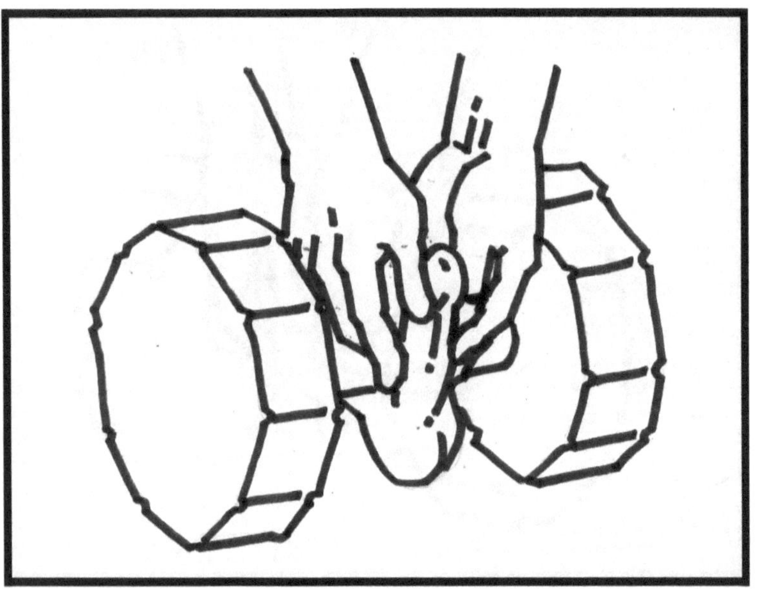

Get your penis in shape as you would your body.

By increasing size and improving erections.
Try penis exercises to enhance your
sex life and self-esteem.

Dedication

This book is dedicated to my brother, Bobby Mike Maxwell, 1954-2004.

NOTE

NOTE

NOTE

NOTE

NOTE

NOTE

NOTE

NOTE

NOTE

NOTE

NOTE

NOTE

NOTE

NOTE

NOTE

NOTE

NOTE

NOTE

NOTE

NOTE

NOTE